STAY FIT ON THE FLY

Managing Weight and Bloating During Travel

by
Elizabeth Miller

Dear Esteemed Reader,

Thank you immensely for choosing this book to join your collection. We imagine that you've already embarked on an exploration of ideas within these pages, and we couldn't be happier about it!

Now, if you find yourself chuckling, pondering, or even debating with the words in front of you, we'd absolutely love to hear about it. If you can spare a few moments to pen down your thoughts in a review, we would be as delighted as a dictionary on a spelling bee!

An Amazon review would be excellent - but hey, we're far from picky. Whether it's a scribble on the back of a grocery list, a tweet, or even a message in a bottle (though that might take a while to reach us), your feedback is gold.

Writing a review might not be as fun as a spontaneous dance-off, but we promise it'll bring grins to our faces, warmth to our hearts, and incredibly valuable insights to future readers.

With Gratitude,

Bo Bennett, PhD
Publisher
Archieboy Holdings, LLC.

Table of Contents

Understanding Your Body:
An Introduction

Let's face it, we've all been there - indulging in airport food, sitting stagnant for long periods on planes, trains, or in cars. Our body feels bloated, sluggish, and overall just plain yucky by the time we hit our destination. But what if it doesn't have to be like that? What if there was a way to feel just as healthy and vibrant as you do when you're at home, even when you're crossing multiple time zones or trying new cuisines?

This book is about helping you get to know your body better, so you can make the best choices while you travel and maintain that feeling of being in balance. We will delve into the basics of gut health and how it impacts not only your waistline, but your overall wellness. We will also take a deep dive into how travelling affects your body and how understanding these effects can make a significant difference to your health during your trips. Simple yet effective strategies to prevent bloating, diet choices, adjusting to your internal body clock, importance of movement and exercising during travel will be discussed too.

We'll also acknowledge the vital connection that your brain has with your body when we cover common travel stressors and their impact. Remember, it's not only what you eat, but also what you think and feel can heavily impact your body. Lastly, we'll not leave you grasping at straws; we'll wrap it up with practical tips to implement these strategies and create a comprehensive travel wellness plan. We hope to give you the guidance you need to keep bloating and weight fluctuations at bay—meaning you can enjoy your work trips or vacations without sacrificing your health goals. So, let's dive in and start your journey to healthier, happier travel!

Chapter 1:
The Basics of Gut Health

L et's dive into it, straight to the heart of the matter: your gut health. You've probably heard the term thrown around in some form or another, but let's lay it bare. When we talk about gut health, we're talking about the array of microorganisms living in your digestive tract- we lovingly call these the gut microbiota. The goal here is balance. If these tiny guests are happy and in harmony, you're likely to have a smoother digestion and less bloating, because your body is handling what you eat efficiently. Conversely, if that harmony is disrupted, it can impact your absorption of nutrients, lead to discomfort and even throw your weight on a wild ride. If your gut health is out of whack, it may very well contribute to those pesky pounds that seem to pop out of nowhere after a trip. So, we can see that understanding our gut health can be one of the keys to keeping our bodies in check while on the move. But don't worry, we're not just throwing facts at you, we've got some concrete steps lined up in the upcoming chapters to make maintaining your gut health more attainable and less of a guessing game.

What Is Gut Health?

Let's dive into the concept of gut health. When we talk about gut health, we're really talking about the multitude of microorganisms, particularly bacteria, that live in our digestive tracts. These organisms, collectively known as the gut microbiota, play an essential role in our overall health. They aid digestion, boost the immune system, produce vitamins, and even influence our behavior and mood.

The state of our gut health can be defined by the balance and diversity of these microorganisms. While we have both 'good' and 'bad' bacteria living in our gut, it's all about maintaining a harmonious balance. Too many 'bad' bacteria, or not enough 'good' bacteria, can lead to health problems. Additionally, the variety of bacteria strains can affect the way we process and store food, which influences body weight and susceptibility to bloating - something we'll delve deeper into later on in the book.

Now, this complex ecosystem can be influenced by a number of factors. Your diet, sleep patterns, stress levels, and even the environment can impact your gut health. In other words, maintaining good gut health requires a comprehensive approach that looks at various aspects of your lifestyle.

While research is ongoing in understanding the ins and outs of gut health, what we do know is that a healthy gut contributes to a strong immune system, heart health, brain health, improved mood, and effective digestion. It may even help prevent some cancers and autoimmune diseases. Doesn't that make you think, right?

Bloating, by the way, is often a sign of a gut that could do with a bit more love. Ever wondered why your stomach feels puffy and hard after a long journey? Or why, as a frequent traveler, you sometimes struggle with bloating? It's often down to disruption in your gut health. When the balance of good and bad bacteria gets thrown off, it can lead to bloating or discomfort.

Another aspect of gut health to consider is something called digestion speed. Basically, this is how quickly food travels through your system. If it's too quick, your body may not be able to absorb all the nutrients, leading to malnutrition, weight loss, and potentially bloating. If it's too slow, food stays in your system for too long, leading to constipation, weight gain, and you guessed it – bloating!

When it comes to gut health and weight fluctuation, they're pretty much partners in crime. You see, imbalanced gut health can lead to weight gain or loss. If the gut isn't processing nutrients effectively due to an imbalance in the gut microbiota, it can lead to either increased or decreased calorie absorption and thus influence weight fluctuation.

Now, this is where it gets particularly interesting for frequent travelers. Every time you take a trip, you expose your body, and therefore your gut microbiota, to a new environment. Everything from the air you breathe to the food you eat can introduce new bacteria into your gut. And guess what? This can impact your gut health.

All this swirl of factors that can affect your gut health does sound a bit overwhelming. But don't fret, there's a lot you can do to maintain a harmonious gut environment, like choosing foods and drinks that foster good bacteria and promote digestion, and trying to maintain healthy stress levels.

We'll look into how you can take charge of factors like food choices, physical activity, and stress management for your gut health in the upcoming sections. And trust me, just a few changes can have a huge impact on enhancing your gut health - and reduce bloating, and weight fluctuation while traveling.

So, proper gut health can be a game-changer in enhancing your overall health and well-being. That's the important key we need to remember. Ensuring our gut is functioning optimally can be a crucial piece in the puzzle of maintaining our health while traveling. So, let's embark on this journey to stronger gut health together, shall we?

And remember, as we navigate this journey to improve gut health while you travel, take it one step at a time. From understanding the role of your gut health to implementing practical tips to maintain it during travel, remember, every small change counts. Don't get overwhelmed, and keep reminding yourself why you're doing it – to ensure your travels are as smooth, comfortable, and healthy as possible.

How Gut Health Affects Weight and Bloating

Your gut is undeniably your second brain. It has a direct influence on your weight and bloating - two issues that can be particularly bothersome while traveling. Let's dive deeper into the intricate relationship between gut health, weight management, and bloating.

The gut, or the gastrointestinal (GI) tract, ferries food from the mouth, via the stomach, and out through the digestive system. So, how your gut functions greatly affects how your body processes fuel, including how fat is stored, blood sugar levels are regulated, and how you metabolically respond to meals.

The ecosystem of bacteria in your gut, known as the gut microbiota, plays a significant role in digestion. Different kinds of bacteria have various roles, and the balance between them can have a massive impact on your health. It's thought that certain bacteria in our guts help us maintain our weight by influencing how we absorb nutrients, and by producing chemicals that help us feel full.

These gut bacteria also impact how dietary fibers are broken down in the body. When fibers are digested by bacteria in your colon, it leads to the production of short-chain fatty acids which are known to aid in weight management.

Consequently, an imbalance of these gut bacteria can adversely affect your weight. Too many undesirable types of bacteria and not enough beneficial bacteria can potentially slow down metabolism and contribute to weight gain. Equally important to note is that traveling can upset this delicate balance due to changes in eating and sleeping patterns.

Now, raise a mental glass of kombucha to your gut, folks! It's working hard for you. If balance is the key, let's delve into how to achieve this inner harmony, especially while being on the move. Taking prebiotics and probiotics can help maintain a healthy balance of gut flora. Your gut microbes also love it when you eat diverse plant-based foods and fiber-rich meals, which can help when trying to manage weight on the go.

Alongside weight, gut health has a considerable effect on bloating. Bloating can result from an overgrowth of gas-producing bacteria in the gut. This overgrowth can be due to consuming certain sugars and carbohydrates that these bacteria thrive on, leading to an increase in gas and a bloated belly.

A quite common condition, namely, Small Intestinal Bacterial Overgrowth (SIBO), can lead to bloating and weight fluctuation. SIBO happens when bacteria from the large intestine move into the small intestine, leading to symptoms like bloating, stomach pain, and weight loss. Remember, this condition requires a medical diagnosis and treatment. If you're frequently bloated or experience severe symptoms, it's a good idea to see a healthcare professional before your journey.

Stress and lack of sleep, often associated with travel, can influence gut health, which, in turn, can exacerbate bloating. Stress can affect gut barrier function, and poor sleep can affect the healthy diversity of gut flora, leading to an increase in harmful bacteria associated with bloating.

All this information might make you feel like walking on eggshells with your gut health. But don't worry. A big part of maintaining a healthy gut, preventing weight gain, and reducing bloating is being mindful of what you feed your gut and how you care for it, especially when traveling.

Eating a balanced diet rich in lean proteins, fruits, vegetables, whole grains, and healthy fats, and drinking plenty of water can help maintain healthy gut flora. Adding fermented foods like yogurt, kefir, and sauerkraut to your diet can also provide beneficial probiotics. Avoiding or limiting consumption of processed foods, high-fat foods, and sugary beverages can also prevent unnecessary weight gain and bloating.

Make a commitment to manage your stress. This can include practicing yoga, meditation, breathing exercises, or anything that effectively helps you relax and unwind. Remember, a calm mind often leads to a happy gut. Also, make it a point to get plenty of sleep. Your gut health and waistline will thank you!

Having a healthy gut isn't just about avoiding weight gain and bloating. It's overall well-being, mental clarity, energy levels, and really, your entire travel experience hinges on it. So, the next time you're packing for a trip, remember to pack yourself some nutritious snacks and consider how you might be able to maintain your gut health while away from home. Your gut will thank you!

Now, go forth and travel knowing a little more about how gut health affects weight and bloating. Remember, when your gut is happy, your travels will be far more comfortable and enjoyable.

Chapter 2:
Traveling and Your Body:
The Impact of Long Journeys

So, we've got the basics down, we understand the good and the bad about gut health, right? Now, let's explore what happens when you decide to step out of your daily routine and embark on a journey. Be it an 8-hour flight, a couple of days on a train, or maybe a cross-country car trip - these long journeys can play tricks on your body that you may not have been aware of. Think about it, during such travel, your body undergoes changes due to factors like prolonged sitting, limited movement, pressure changes, and let's not overlook the nutritional impact of grabbing fast food or airplane snacks when healthier options are tough to find. Some common unpleasant experiences include dehydration, bloating, tiredness, and even swelling of the feet. Sure, it doesn't sound all that appealing, but understanding these effects, that's the key. With knowledge of how your body is likely to react, you can take small yet significant steps to manage and even prevent some of these issues. That's what we're after - making sure that your much-anticipated travel doesn't turn into a health nightmare. So, let's unpack the effects that different modes of travel can have on your body, and then, using the wonders of science, we're going to arm ourselves with enough knowledge to fight off the biggest travel health culprits. A bit of knowledge and preparation, my friend, could make all the difference to your travel experience.

The Effects of Flying on Your Body

You've just wrapped up your last meeting and it's finally time to head home. You're sitting in the airport, waiting for your flight, wondering how this journey may affect your body. Is your waistline going to expand with every time zone crossed? Is a cocktail of bloating, weight fluctuation and general discomfort waiting for you as you disembark?

Challenges like these are just part of the many effects of the flying experience. Let's dive into the physiological changes that occur while you're in the air. This will help you understand how you can lessen their impacts during your travels.

Firstly, the low humidity of the cabin air in most commercial flights can quickly lead to dehydration. This dry environment causes your body to lose water at a faster rate than usual. And, don't forget, dehydration can induce feelings of fatigue and exacerbate symptoms of jet lag, which we'll touch on later.

Alongside dehydration, the reduced air pressure and oxygen levels at high altitudes can sometimes lead to a condition known as 'altitude sickness'. When this happens, you may experience dizziness, nausea, and headaches.

Bloating is another common issue you may face whilst flying. Because of the lower pressure at high altitudes, gas in your body expands. This gas expansion cause you to feel bloated and could even lead to stomach discomfort.

These aren't the only effects though, you're also more likely to catch a cold or flu on a plane. Long flights particularly, keep you in close quarters with several other passengers for an extended period, increasing the chance of catching an airborne virus. So, keep hand sanitizer handy and don't hesitate to use it frequently.

How about that notorious jet lag? The rapid crossing of multiple time zones disrupts your body's internal clock, leading to this disorienting and energy-sapping phenomenon known as jet lag. Jet lag can cause fatigue, insomnia, gastrointestinal problems, and even mild depression until your body adjusts to the new time zone.

So how about some good news? Indeed flying can also have a few positive effects on your body. An airplane's cabin pressure can actually reduce symptoms of certain chronic respiratory disorders. Also psychologically, the idea of traveling can boost your mood and quench your thirst for discovery which can indirectly improve your overall health.

It's also worth noting that immobilization for long periods of time, like during a long-haul flight, can increase the risk of developing deep vein thrombosis (DVT). This condition is caused when blood clots form, typically in the legs, due to poor circulation. This is a serious condition that requires immediate medical attention.

The impact of flying on your body can be minimized by engaging in regular movement during the flight. Stand, stretch and walk up and down the aisle when it's safe to do so. This can help stimulate circulation and reduce the risk of developing DVT.

Combating the dehydrating effect of low cabin humidity can also be achieved by sipping on water throughout the journey. Remember to avoid alcohol and caffeine, which can further dehydrate you.

While the plane's cabin pressure can lead to bloating, eating light meals and avoiding gas-producing foods can help mitigate this uncomfortable sensation.

Lastly, encourage your body to acclimate more quickly to time zone changes by adjusting your watch to the time zone of your destination as soon as you board. Try to stay awake during the day and sleep at night according to the new time zone. This can help your body adjust faster and reduce the effects of jet lag.

In conclusion, while flying can certainly have a profound effect on your body, being armed with understanding and a few handy tips can make all the difference. By implementing these practices, you'll not only feel better during and after your flight, but also stay healthy and refresh as you cross those time zones.

Car and Train Travel: What's Happening to Your Body?

Imagine you're on a road trip, or perhaps you're on a train whizzing past beautiful landscapes. It's easy to get lost in the journey's excitement and forget about our body's needs. But, the thing is, car and train travel impact you physically, often in surprising ways.

Firstly, let's chat about sitting. For many, traveling via car or train means a heap of time spent sitting. Though it gives our legs a break, sitting for prolonged periods can increase the risk of developing heart disease, diabetes, and other health conditions. It can also lead to unnecessary weight gain and bloating. Plus, because circulation tends to decrease when we're sitting, there's the risk of deep vein thrombosis (DVT), particularly on longer journeys.

Now, let's consider the snacks. When you're traveling by road or rail, it's tempting to indulge in the comfort of fast foods, sugary drinks, and snack foods. Comfort food has a place for nostalgia or as an occasional treat, but leaning on it can lead to bloating and unhealthy weight gain.

Here's a key insight: it's not just about what you eat, but how you eat as well. When we're gnawing on snacks absent-mindedly while watching the world go by, we often eat faster and chew less. This can result in swallowing air (the culprit behind bloating) and overeating too.

Dehydration is another concern on long car or train rides. It might not seem intuitive, but being confined within an air-conditioned vehicle can be dehydrating. Reduced fluid intake to minimize bathroom breaks, the presence of sugary or caffeinated drinks, and a dry environment contribute to this. As we know, dehydration isn't great - it can lead to headaches, feeling tired, and even impact digestion.

Here's a big one - stress. Travel, as thrilling as it is, can trigger stress hormones in our bodies. When we're trying to navigate traffic or catching tight connections, our bodies respond by entering 'fight-or-flight' mode, robust from our prehistoric ancestors. It meant survival back then. But now? It can lead to both immediate and long-term health issues, including weight gain and increased bloating.

Plus, our bowel movements can be affected when we're on the go. Strange toilets, tight schedules, or just being in an unfamiliar environment can lead to irregularity. Let's not forget, disrupted sleep patterns due to long travel days or late-night rides can impact our bodies' metabolism, potentially leading to weight changes and bloating.

So, yeah, traveling isn't always a walk in the park for our bodies. But don't ditch your travel plans just yet!

Understanding these factors is a huge step toward mitigating their effects. Simple adjustments can bring palpable relief. Like, take regular breaks during your journey to stretch, move, and stimulate blood flow. It refreshes your mind, reduces the risk of DVT, and lets you enjoy the journey a bit more.

Meal planning could be your new best friend, and sticking to wholesome, homemade meals or healthy options can keep those snack cravings at bay, maintaining weight and reducing bloating. To stay hydrated, make water your go-to, and don't resist those bathroom breaks!

Managing stress through calming activities like listening to your favorite playlist or an absorbing audiobook can do wonders. And building a routine, no matter how brief your journey is, can help normalize sleep patterns and meal times, keeping your metabolism and digestion on track.

Lastly, listen to your body. Each of us reacts differently to travel. What works for one person might not work for another. Identify the situations and foods that bother you and adjust accordingly.

Train or car journeys, long or short, should be a time of enjoyment and discovery, not discomfort. Armed with a better understanding of what's happening to your body, you can transform your travel experiences into healthier ones. By making some conscious, mindful decisions during your journey, you can ensure that your body doesn't bear the brunt of your wanderlust.

Facts About the Human Body and Travel As we continue our exploration of how travel and health intertwine, we can't ignore the quite fascinating nuggets of information on the impact of travel on our bodies. When you're sitting on a plane bumping along at 36,000 feet, something weird happens in your intestines. The changes in cabin pressure can cause gases to expand in the gut, leading to bloating. It's no wonder you feel a little extra uncomfortable after a long flight. Also, the reduction in oxygen at high altitudes might make digestion less efficient, exacerbating that bloated feeling, hence it's not only about that second airplane snack you can't resist.

It's not just in-flight issues we're talking about here. Let's consider jet lag. It's your body's response to rapid changes in time zones. Sure, in theory, you've traveled to a new destination in just a matter of hours. But unfortunately, your circadian rhythms—the natural internal process that regulates the sleep-wake cycle every 24 hours—hasn't been equally quick to adapt. It still thinks you're back home, leading to a range of unpleasant manifestations including fatigue, sleep disturbance, and yep, you guessed it — bloating.

And finally, here's an interesting twist. Travel isn't all bad news. Hopping on a plane can actually be good for the heart (literally!). When we're in the air, the heart doesn't have to work as hard to pump blood upwards, making it a mini vacation for the most important muscle in your body. Isn't that something? But before you get too excited, this doesn't mean you should skip your regular exercises. A healthy travel lifestyle needs an all-round approach, so keep that in mind next time you're planning your trip.

How Understanding Science Can Help You Stay Fit and Healthy The beauty of science is that it can be incredibly practical, especially when it comes to understanding your body and keeping it healthy. A strong grasp of scientific principles can be your best ally when it comes to staying fit while traveling. It doesn't mean you have to dust off your high school biology textbook, but rather understanding simple aspects like the body's reaction to physical stress or difference in altitudes can provide you with an edge in maintaining your health while on the road.

First off, it's important to understand how physical stress, like travel, impacts your body. Long flights, for instance, can lead to jet lag, the nagging fatigue that follows as a mixed cocktail of extended sitting, cabin air, and disrupted sleep. This exhaustion can, in turn, throw off your entire body system - your digestion, metabolism, mental clarity, and so much more. By understanding the science behind these shifts, it's easier to prepare and manage it effectively when it happens.

Let's break down another large aspect - hydration. Everybody knows that it's essential to stay hydrated, especially while traveling. But do you know why? It's because water acts as a transport system within your body, moving nutrients around, eliminating waste, and maintaining the optimum body temperature. Airplane cabins are extremely dry and can lead to quick dehydration, causing that dreaded travel fatigue and even sometimes resulting in you feeling bloated.

And speaking of bloating, the science of your gut health plays a huge role here too. The balance of good and bad bacteria in your gut, also known as gut microbiota, largely determines how your body stores fat, balances glucose levels, and responds to hormones that make you feel hungry or full. Traveling, due to irregular eating and sleeping patterns, can disrupt this sensitive environment, resulting in bloating or weight gain. By being attentive to what you're eating while on the go, you can keep your gut bacteria balanced and happy.

Finally, comprehension of your circadian rhythm, or your body's internal clock, can work wonders. This complex science dictates when you feel sleepy, hungry, or energetic. It is incredibly influenced by light exposure, meals, and social engagement. Flying across time zones can throw your rhythm off, causing sleeplessness, digestive issues, or sluggishness. But by gradually adjusting your sleep, meal, and social schedules to the new time zone prior to traveling, you can significantly reduce the impact on your circadian rhythm.

By leaning into the science behind the body and travel, you're setting yourself up for a healthier and more enjoyable journey. Sure, maintaining your health while traveling can seem like a tricky puzzle, but with a bit of knowledge and the right preparations, it doesn't have to be!

Chapter 3:
Your Body's Internal Clock:
Adjusting to New Time Zones

Let's switch gears and talk about your body's internal clock, your circadian rhythm. The circadian rhythm, our body's biological timepiece, manages numerous physiological functions, including sleep-wake cycles, feeding habits, digestion, and immunity. You see, when you fly from New York to London - just for instance - your body still retains its original schedule. It's like that song that's stuck in your head on repeat. So, the result? You're wide awake when you should be sleeping, hungry when it's not mealtime, and your digestion process might as well have been handed bingo numbers. Here's a tip, start adjusting to your destination's time zone before you leave. Move your meals, your bedtime, even your Netflix watching schedule ahead (or behind) an hour or two. Sounds simple, sure, but trust me, it's a game-changer. Doing this, gradually, can help recalibrate your internal clock to the new time zone, so your body doesn't feel like it's on the wrong side of a musical chair game. But we'll have more on that, and some other cool science-based strategies for your travel toolkit, in a bit.

Understanding Circadian Rhythms

As travelers, we experience changes in time zones that can affect our body's natural clock, commonly referred to as our circadian rhythm. Maybe you've heard that phrase before or maybe not, but let's go ahead and delve deeper into this term to truly understand what it means.

Quite simply, circadian rhythms are the natural physical, mental, and behavioral changes within a 24-hour cycle that respond primarily to light and darkness in your environment. They play a massive role in your sleep-wake cycle, feeding times, body temperature, and various other physiological processes. Getting a grasp on your personal circadian rhythm can provide an advantage when managing the effects of time changes while traveling.

Your internal body clock affects the production of melatonin, which is the hormone responsible for making you sleepy at night. When it gets dark, more melatonin gets produced, encouraging sleep. Conversely, sunshine results in a decrease in melatonin production, encouraging wakefulness. That's why a sunny morning makes you feel more awake and alert.

Now, here's the kicker: traveling across different time zones interrupts that beautiful rhythm. The sudden change of light and darkness can confuse our circadian rhythm, which in turn affects our sleep, eating habits, and even bowel movements. Yes, that adds to the bloating too. This is what's commonly known as jet lag.

Think of your body as a orchestra where your circadian rhythm is like the conductor. For the orchestra to make harmonious music, all the instruments (or in our case, physiological processes) need to follow the conductor's direction. If the conductor is offbeat or missing, the music becomes discordant. The same goes for our bodies when our circadian rhythm gets thrown off by travel.

It's worth noting that everyone's circadian rhythm can slightly vary, with some people often dubbed as 'night owls' or 'morning larks'. A 'night owl' tends to feel more energetic in the later part of the day while 'morning larks' wake up bright and cheery at sunrise. Conveniently, these natural sleep patterns can be leveraged when traveling across different time zones, but more on that later.

Your circadian rhythm doesn't just govern your sleep-wake cycle, it also plays a part in hunger, digestion, and metabolism. Recent research suggests that our body even reacts to food differently at various times of the day because of our internal body clock. That's why you might feel famished after a red-eye flight or experience constipation or bloating when traveling across multiple time zones. Sound familiar?

The good news is, one can train and adjust their circadian rhythm towards a new time zone, which essentially reduces the impact of jet lag. Gradual adjustment to the time zone you're traveling to can start even before you leave your home. It predominantly involves adjusting your sleep schedule and exposure to light.

And here's another golden nugget: exercise regulated according to your destination time zone can help in adapting your circadian rhythm. Regular physical activity triggers your body to adjust to new 'awake' and 'rest' periods. Timing your exercise according to your new time zone can train your body clock faster. We'll discuss more about this in the coming chapters.

It's also worth pointing out that artificial blue light emitted by digital screens can disrupt your circadian rhythm by suppressing melatonin production. So, cutting back on screen time, especially in the evenings, can help maintain a regular sleep-wake cycle.

Understanding circadian rhythms may seem like something out of a school science textbook, but it is undeniably important for maintaining physical health, especially when traveling. Remember, the more you know about how your body works, the better you can adjust and make decisions that will help you avoid bloating and assist your general wellbeing as you trot around the globe.

How Travelling across Time Zones Affects Your Body

Moving between time zones can mess with your body's rhythm big time. It's more than just the annoyance of having to reset your wristwatch; your internal biological clock needs a reset too, and it often doesn't happen as easily.

The primary effect of crossing time zones is a temporary disorder famously known as jet lag. It's your body's loud and clear reaction, telling you that something doesn't seem right. You feel sleepy when it's broad daylight, and unfortunately wide awake when it feels like bedtime. This is because your body's internal clock is struggling to adjust to the new time zone.

It starts with the hypothalamus: it's this part of your brain that controls your circadian rhythm. As you are traveling across time zones, your exposure to light changes. Since your hypothalamus uses light to control sleep patterns, meal times, and other bodily functions, it becomes all jumbled up. It's like your brain is living in New York, but your body has landed in Los Angeles.

But that's not where the effects end. You know how when you're on a long flight, you feel like there's a balloon in your gut? Yeah, that's the effect of the change in time zones on your digestive system. Your body remains on its original schedule for a few days, so you might feel hungry at odd timings.

This misalignment can lead to various symptoms of jet lag like fatigue, difficulty concentrating, disorientation, irritability, nausea, and even mild depression. Jet lag can be tough, especially when you need to be in top form for an important meeting or an adventurous travel itinerary.

However, the severity of this time zone change's effect can vary based on the direction of travel. Most people find it harder when traveling east rather than west. This is because we are essentially "losing time" when we travel east, making it difficult for our bodies to adapt, kind of like trying to fall asleep when you're not quite tired.

Apart from direction, the number of time zones crossed is another factor that influences how your body reacts. The more time zones you cross during your journey, the more severe and prolonged are the potential effects.

Don't worry, it's not all doom and gloom, and your body can certainly adjust to the new time zone. It roughly takes about one day per time zone for your body to adapt. So, if you've crossed three time zones, your body should be good to go after about three days. But let's be honest, who's got that much time to waste when you're traveling?

Another physical impact is the potential for fluid retention, aka, bloating. This could be due to sitting for long hours on a plane, but the change in the circadian rhythm also plays its part. It may lead you to eat or drink at uneven intervals, causing your body to retain more fluid than usual.

Frequent travelers may also experience menstrual irregularities due to traveling across time zones. Women's menstrual cycles are regulated by a complex hormonal orchestra that can be sensitive to changes in time zones. A disruption in the normal sleep/wake cycle can send signals to the hormonal system to delay or advance the menstrual cycle.

Understanding how traveling across time zones affects the body is the first step to mitigating these effects. It's absolutely fine to indulge in the occasional afternoon power nap, eat a healthy meal when you feel hungry, even if it's not mealtime yet, and, very importantly, try to adapt to local time as quickly as possible.

Remember, these time-change symptoms are short-term and your body is rather amazing at adjusting to new environments. The real goal here is to take care of yourself during this adjustment phase. Only then will you truly be able to enjoy your travels without constantly battling your own body.

Last but not least, it's important to scientifically align your sleep cycle with the destination time zone even before starting your journey. Adjust your bedtime, wakeup time, and meals according to the new time zone a couple of days before you're set to jet off. This might not wipe out jet lag entirely, but it can certainly help to lessen the symptoms and make the adjustment process smoother.

Chapter 4:
Healthy Eating for Travel:
Foods to Prevent Bloating

Heading into our latest topic, let's hone in on what we can do to prevent bloating issues while we're on the move. Remember the science we've been diving into about your gut health and how travel can throw it off-balance? Yup, it's time to apply that knowledge into your meal choices. So, what's causing the bloating? Well, there's a laundry list of potential culprits but a common offender is our food choices. High sodium foods exacerbate bloating by making your body hold onto excess water. Simple carbohydrates, like white bread or pastries, can also leave you feeling bloated. Consuming these while sitting for extended periods during long haul travel is a recipe for discomfort. On the flip side, foods rich in potassium (think bananas, avocados, spinach) can combat puffiness by balancing out sodium levels. Foods high in fiber, such as whole grains, beans and peas, fruits and vegetables, will help keep your digestive system running smoothly. Just remember to ease into a high-fiber diet, too much too fast can backfire and lead to bloating. Probiotic foods like yogurt and kimchi can help restore gut balance, potentially reducing bloating and promoting overall digestive health. And let's not forget hydration - water aids digestion and can help curb bloating by flushing out your system. Remember that balance is key, and what works for you may be different from others, so pay close attention to your body's reaction to different foods. It may take some tweaking to find the right mix that works for you, but it's a worthwhile journey.

What Causes Bloating?

Picture this—there you are, hovering thirty thousand feet in the air, cramped between dodgy airplane food trays and the unyielding arms of your seat. Suddenly, your jeans start to feel a tad bit tight. Your belly feels swollen, and you're uncomfortably distended. That, my friends, is the dreaded bloating.

Bloating is an uncomfortable feeling of fullness in the abdominal area, often accompanied by distention. While it's normal to experience some bloating after a big meal, frequent bloating could signal an underlying issue that needs to be addressed. So, the real question is, what causes bloating?

Let's start with food—after all, we are what we eat. Certain foods are renowned for causing gas and bloating, such as beans, onions, broccoli, cabbage, sprouts, and carbonated drinks. When these are consumed in large amounts, especially combined with a sedentary lifestyle like prolonged sitting during air travel, they contribute significantly to bloating. The digestive system can't break them down completely, so gas builds up in the stomach, causing bloating.

Next up is dehydration. If you're not taking in enough fluids, especially water, your body tends to hold onto the water it does have, creating a bloated feeling. This happens a lot during air travel because the humidity inside an airplane is typically lower than we're accustomed to, which can lead to dehydration. So, if you're not sipping on lots of water, you might be making more room for bloating.

Speed eating is another common culprit when it comes to bloating. When you eat quickly, you're likely swallowing air along with your food. This causes gas to build inside your digestive tract, leading to bloating. Add the factor of eating on the go, which often means not chewing each bite properly, and it's a recipe for a bloated belly.

Another contributor to bloating is a disruption in your gut microbes. Your gut is home to trillions of tiny microbes that help digest your food, but travel can disrupt this delicate ecosystem. Jet lag, changes in diet, and general travel-induced stress can mess with your gut microbes, leading to bloating and other gastrointestinal disturbances.

Surprisingly enough, your dinner can be a major bloating culprit, as well. Large meals are harder for your system to digest, and when they combine with other bloating triggers, like air swallowing or eating gas-producing foods, they can lead to severe bloating.

Don't underestimate the role of stress either! Stress or changes in routine, both of which are inevitable during travel, can wreak havoc on your digestive system. When you're stressed, your body diverts resources away from digestion to other critical functions, leaving undigested food to ferment and cause bloating.

Speaking of diversion, restrictive clothing is another bloating culprit. Skinny jeans or tight belts can compress your stomach and intestines, disrupting the natural digestion process, causing gas to build up, and inducing bloating.

Lastly, certain medications and health issues can cause bloating. If you're taking medication that lists bloating as a side effect, or if you have a medical condition that causes bloating, such as irritable bowel syndrome (IBS) or gastroesophageal reflux disease (GERD), then you may be more prone to bloating during your travels.

It's important to remember that everyone's body is different, so what causes bloating in one person might not be the culprit for someone else. The causes we've mentioned here are fairly universal, but it's always wise to listen to your body and observe how different foods and lifestyle changes affect you personally.

By understanding what triggers bloating, we can start to take steps to alleviate the discomfort and prevent it from happening. In the following sections, we'll dive into food choices that can help reduce bloating during travel. So, sit tight (not too tight, though, we don't want to contribute to bloating), and let's journey further into the realm of maintaining gut health while on the move.

Food Choices to Reduce Bloating During Travel

To stay bloating-free throughout your journey, it's critical to be mindful of your food choices. What you consume before and during travel plays a crucial role in your overall health and comfort. Now, let's travel through the terrain of food choices that can lessen bloating during your sojourns.

Firstly, consider vegetables and fruits as your travel companions. They are high in fiber and improve digestion, reducing the potential for bloating. Opt for fruits like blueberries, oranges, or pineapples, which have high water content and can keep you hydrated. As for veggies, lean towards cucumbers, zucchinis, and bell peppers that are packed with water and nutrients. Just remember to go easy as excessive fiber can sometimes cause bloating if your body isn't used to it.

At the same time, pay heed to the proteins you're packing in your diet. Low-fat proteins such as chicken, turkey, or fish are excellent choices. They provide necessary nutrition without increasing the chances of bloating as saturated fats can. Also, consider plant-based proteins such as lentils or tofu, but again, if your body isn't accustomed to these, introducing them slowly is key.

A handful of nuts or seeds can also help curb your hunger without causing bloating. Almonds, walnuts, and flaxseeds are perfect travel snacks. They're rich in fiber and healthy fats, filling your stomach while keeping it flat.

It might be tempting to reach for a bag of chips or some cookies while you're on the go, but the excess sodium and sugars in these processed foods can lead to water retention and bloating. Instead, pack healthier snack alternatives like kale chips, apple slices, or homemade trail mix with dried fruits and nuts.

Beverages also play a crucial role in bloating control. Keep caffeinated drinks and alcohol to a minimum. Sure, a cup of coffee or a glass of wine won't hurt, but overconsumption can lead to dehydration, eventually causing bloating and discomfort. Green tea or hot water with lemon can be a cleaner alternative to combat bloating on the go.

Now, you may be wondering, 'What about bread and pasta?' While these staples might be tempting, they contain refined carbohydrates that could contribute to bloating. Instead, replace these with whole-grain alternatives. Whole grains are less likely to cause bloating as they contain more fiber and make you feel full faster.

Avoid consuming carbonated drinks as they place extra gas in your stomach, which can lead to bloating. Stick to flat water, herbal teas, or freshly squeezed fruit juice as your main sources of fluid. A little-known tip is to drink from a cup or glass instead of a bottle to reduce the ingestion of air bubbles which can add to the bloating phenomenon.

Sometimes, gas and bloating can also result from eating large meals. To avoid this, consider eating more frequent, smaller meals throughout your travel day. This helps to maintain steady blood sugar levels, keeps hunger at bay, and reduces the chances of overeating which can cause bloating.

Dairy can be another bloating culprit, especially for those who are lactose intolerant. If you tend to bloat after eating dairy products, it might be beneficial to look into alternatives like almond milk, coconut yogurt, or lactose-free cheeses during travel.

Eating out while traveling is part of the experience, but it can also contribute to bloating if you're not mindful of what you order. To avoid excess sodium and oil, which can lead to water retention and bloating, opt for grilled or baked proteins, plenty of colorful vegetables, and steer clear of heavy, cream-based sauces.

Fermented foods are also great for gut health which plays an important role in bloating. Foods like kefir, sauerkraut, and kimchi contain probiotics that encourage healthy gut bacteria. But, since these foods can be an acquired taste and may need refrigeration, it's not necessary to force them into your travel diet – just consider incorporating them into your diet in the long term for their benefits.

In a nutshell, staying bloating-free while traveling doesn't need to be complicated. With smart food and beverage choices and a bit of planning, you can ensure that bloating doesn't become an unwelcome travel companion. The bottom line is, understand your body, listen to it, and cater to its needs by providing it with wholesome and nutritious options.

Remember, good nutrition is not just about eating healthy on the road; it's also about feeling good and enjoying your trip to the fullest. Here's to happy and 'bloat-free' travels!

Chapter 5:
Keeping Fit: The Importance of Exercise During Travel

While traveling, the temptation to kick back and neglect your fitness can be overwhelming, but incorporating regular exercise into your travel routine is crucial. It's easy to let the thrill of new adventures sweep you off your feet—literally—but it's important to remember that keeping active isn't just about maintaining a trim waistline. In fact, regular exercise can greatly improve your gut health, boosting your metabolism and lessening the bloating that often follows long trips. On top of that, it aids in regulating your circadian rhythm, thus helping you combat the effects of jet lag. Simple exercises, like brisk walks or short jogs, light yoga, or low-intensity bodyweight exercises, can fit quite seamlessly into your travel itinerary. You don't have to hit the gym hard; just aim for at least 30 minutes of physical activity daily, and you'll notice a stark difference in how you feel. For those long haul flights? Try to stand and stretch every hour; it does wonders for your circulation and will significantly reduce overall feelings of discomfort. As a friendly reminder: exercise should never feel like a chore. See it as a way of exploring new terrain or a chance to unwind. Overall, keeping fit while traveling doesn't just sustain your physical health—it also boosts your mood and increases your energy levels, helping you make the most of every journey.

Why Exercise Matters

So, we've landed at this all-important question: why does exercise matter on your journeys? Whether you're a frequent flier or a casual traveler, physical activity should be high on your agenda. And not just because it reduces bloating (though that's a significant bonus!).

Exercise impacts virtually every aspect of your bodily function. From mind to muscles, heart to hormone production—everything gets a beneficial boost when you stay active. Calories are burned, energy levels are boosted, mood-enhancing endorphins are released, and your immune system gets a much-needed pick-me-up. With your body running like a well-oiled machine, bloating becomes less of an issue, even in the cramped conditions of a plane or car.

Now, stopping at a gym while jetting from place to place may seem impossible (and quite frankly, it's not on everyone's top-ten list of vacation activities). But the good news is, you don't have to! Simple exercises and mindful movement can keep your body ticking over nicely, even if you have a busy schedule or you're stuck in your seat on a long flight.

Let's say you're on a transatlantic flight for hours. This extended period of inactivity slows your metabolism, reduces blood circulation, and may amplify bloating. Just by doing small activities like rotating your ankles, stretching your arms, or doing body twists intermittently can make a significant difference. These exercises can stimulate blood flow and kick-start your metabolism, helping to prevent or reduce bloating.

If you're traveling by train or planning a road-trip, you have even more options. During pitstops or at stations, you can squeeze in some quick activities like lunges, squats, or even a brisk walk. This not only wakes up your muscles but it also makes you feel more alert and less sluggish.

Another great idea is going for a jog or stroll to explore the new city you're visiting. This provides the dual benefits of sightseeing and easy yet effective exercise. Just remember to keep your pace brisk enough to get your heart rate up!

The benefits of exercise don't stop at a fit body. It's a well-documented fact that regular physical activity has huge perks for mental health. Exercise releases mood-boosting chemicals like endorphins and serotonin, which can leave you feeling happier, more relaxed, and less stressed. Given the unfamiliarity and potential challenges of travel, this mental boost can be a game changer in managing travel-related anxiety or stress.

Let's talk about jet lag now. Crossing time zones can wreak havoc on your body clock, disrupting your sleep and leaving you feeling fatigued, disoriented, and generally out of sorts. Regular exercise can help you reset your internal clock faster. Science has shown that working out can actually shift your body's circadian rhythm, helping to speed up that adjustment to new time zones.

Travel should be enjoyable, fulfilling, and revitalizing. Long periods of inactivity, poor diet choices, and stress, however, often get in the way of that ideal. We can't always control our environment when we're on the move, but we do have power over our lifestyle choices. Prioritizing workouts, even light ones, can be a transformative choice that promotes your physical well-being and enriches your travel experience.

So, the next time your travel planner is out, leave some space for physical activity right alongside those must-see sights or important business meetings. It's not just about maintaining your fitness level; it's also a recipe for more vibrant health, greater energy, better mood, less bloating, and overall, a much more enjoyable experience on the road.

By now, you might be thinking, "Okay, I get it, exercising is important. But what kind of exercises are we talking about?". No worries, we've got you covered in the next section with simple but effective exercises you can do while traveling. So, let's start infusing fitness into your travel plans, shall we?

Simple Exercises for the Traveller

Carrying on from the importance of exercise as we discussed earlier, let's delve into more specific exercises for you, our health-conscious travelers.

Long journeys can mess up your regular workout routines. So, the key is to stick to simple exercises that require little or no equipment and can be done in small spaces. Plane aisles, train compartments, or hotel rooms, bring it on! Here are a few simple exercises that you can easily incorporate into your travel itinerary.

1. Walking

Walking is a simple and effective exercise that doesn't need any special equipment. Explore new cities on foot, choose the stairs instead of the elevator, or just take a brisk walk around your hotel. Not only is walking great for your heart health, but it can also keep bloating at bay.

2. Stretching

Stretching exercises are easy to perform and can be done basically anywhere. Whether you're on a long flight or in your hotel room, incorporate simple stretches in your routine to improve flexibility and reduce muscle discomfort from those long hours of sitting.

3. Body weight exercises

Your own body weight can be your best fitness tool. Think push-ups, squats, lunges, and planks. These exercises require minimal space and can be performed in your hotel room. They can help strengthen your core, improve balance and fight off those extra travel calories.

4. Yoga

Yoga can be a great travel workout tool. A few sun salutations in your hotel room or a vinyasa flow at a local park can work wonders. It calms the mind, balances the body and can help you adjust better to new time zones.

5. Using a resistance band

Can't leave behind your love for strength training? A resistance band is your answer. It's lightweight, portable, and can help you in working out different muscle groups. Perfect for performing strength training exercises in the confines of your hotel room.

Remember, the best workout is the one you'll stick with. So, pick what you enjoy most and fit it into your travel schedule. If you love running, find local parks or tracks. A fitness enthusiast? Look for a local gym.

It's essential not to turn these workouts into another stress factor. They're meant to be flexible and adapted according to your travel schedule. Missed a workout because of a late-night flight? No problem. Just pick it up the next day. It's about consistency and not perfection.

Certainly, exercising during travel can ensure your body remains active and healthy, aiding digestion and reducing bloating. More than that, it enables you to continue your fitness journey, no matter where you are, ensuring a proactive and positive trip.

The beauty is in the simplicity of these workouts, which makes them achievable. Plus, they could turn a rather dull or stressful travel day into a productive and even enjoyable one! Remember, the view from a mountain top is far better enjoyed after a good climb!

In this way, you'll be better able to keep yourself fit, trim, and ready to fully enjoy your travel experiences, without the specter of bloating or unwanted weight gain looming over you. So, pack your workout gear, and make your next trip a healthy one!

Chapter 6:
How Your Brain Impacts Your Body

Moving on from our previous conversations about our bodies, let's turn our spotlight to the upstairs segment - our brain. It's pretty amazing to think that this three-pound organ controls our health, right? When we're on the go, navigating through airports, cramming ourselves into economy seats or roadside rooms, our brain is impacted - stress tends to skyrocket, and spoiler alert - it can have a real effect on our bodies. What sorts of effects, you ask? Well, too much stress can lead to bloating, weight gain, and low energy levels. Remember those long-term stress hormones we discussed a few chapters back? When your body is constantly stressed, it pumps out cortisol, which can lead to weight gain. Stress can also muddle with your gut, causing you to feel bloated or uncomfortable. No, it's not your imagination; your jet-lagged brain really is influencing your body! But don't fret, keeping calm and collected while traveling is a skill you can develop, and as a bonus, your body will thank you for it.

Common Stressors While Traveling

Traveling can open a world of opportunity, excitement, and curiosity for many individuals. However, with these adventures can come a series of stressors that might challenge your mental and physical wellbeing. First and foremost, let's talk about the anxiety surrounding the anticipation of the trip itself. You're probably double-checking your packing, coordinating transportation, wrapping up your work, and managing numerous tasks before setting off, and this can invariably spike your stress levels.

Then, there's the uncertainty factor. Not knowing exactly what's ahead, or not having control over your usual environment, can make you feel uneasy. This can be particularly potent if you're heading to an unfamiliar destination. Uncertainty can stir up a level of anxiety, leading to increased stress and potential discomfort in your body, such as bloating and weight fluctuation.

Next, let's talk about travel logistics. This can include flight delays, lost luggage, navigation troubles, traffic jams, and more. These inconveniences can send your stress levels soaring, and your brain responds by setting off the stress response, which can put your body in a state of heightened tension.

Additionally, there's the impact of changing time zones and disrupting your regular circadian rhythm. Your sleep cycles can easily be out of sync when traveling across time zones, and the resulting jet lag can induce stress. It disrupts your routine and can cause irritability, trouble focusing, and general unrest, all contributing to extra pressure on your body.

Let's not forget the potential of travelling with others. While companionship is often welcome, different personalities, preferences, and pace can cause intersocial stress. This can range from minor disagreements over activities to scheduling clashes and personal space issues, leading to both mental and physical tension.

Then there are the health-related worries such as eating out more, which can impact your diet and exercise routine. You might worry about gaining weight, experiencing bloating, or falling off your fitness plan. This stressor can be particularly noticeable for those conscious about maintaining their health while traveling.

Exposure to new environments can also lead to potential health risks such as food poisoning or exposure to unfamiliar bacteria and viruses, which can lead to heightened stress and anxiety about health and safety. Not to mention the fear of losing your essential items, like passports, wallets, or mobile devices. These unexpected events are not uncommon when traveling and can cause significant stress.

Work-related stress is another factor worth mentioning. If you're traveling for work, there might be presentations, meetings, or business negotiations that bring about their own level of stress. Even if you're on vacation, you might be worried about the pile of work waiting for you when you get back, which can constantly keep you on edge.

Social stressors, such as language barriers, cultural differences, or social norms in a new environment, can also create anxiety. It can be challenging and stressful to connect and communicate effectively in a new cultural setting, which can contribute to overall stress levels.

The conundrum of maintaining good gut health while traveling is a also major stressor. The uncertainties about accessing healthy food choices, the temptation of local cuisines which may not always align with your regular diet, or the fear of food poisoning, could all add to the stress.

Budget constraints may also amplify stress. Fretting over costs, adhering to a budget, or dealing with unforeseen expenses can induce stress, disrupting your heart rate, sleep patterns, and even digestion.

Despite all these stressors, let's face it, traveling is full of beautiful moments and experiences that outweigh the stress. And acknowledging these common stressors is the first step. Once you're aware of what can potentially trigger stress, you're well on your way to managing, if not overcoming, these challenges. The next step is to dive deep into understanding how stress, especially when traveling, impacts your body, and how you can stay physically healthy even when on the go.

Remember, stressors are not all sinister. They simply offer us the chance to adapt and become more resilient travelers. They teach us to stay open, flexible, grounded, and healthy, no matter where our journeys take us. And they provide us with the opportunity to take care of our physical bodies, owing to our mental resilience.

The key takeaway? Know the common travel stressors, understand that they are common and you're not alone in experiencing them. Moreover, realize the profound influence of your brain's reaction to these stressors on your body's response. With this knowledge, you're already on your way to happier, healthier, stress-reduced travel. The journey continues as we delve into exploring how exactly our brains can affect our bodies following the response to stress. The exciting voyage of understanding awaits...

Facts About How the Human Brain can Affect Your Body When Stressed

We've all experienced the feeling of stress: that pounding heart, the sweaty palms, and that sense of urgency. But how exactly does stress affect our bodies, particularly when we're away from home and traveling?

When you're dealing with unfamiliar surroundings or complications, such as delayed flights, lost luggage, or language barriers, your brain goes into overdrive trying to manage all these unexpected stressors. This can lead to various physical reactions that can be particularly problematic for frequent travelers.

So buckle down, because we're about to delve into the ways your brain can affect your body when you're feeling stressed, particularly during travel.

Under stress, the human brain activates what's called the fight or flight response. This basically means your brain starts producing hormones like adrenaline and cortisol to help you react to perceived threats. It's this reaction that can lead to those stress-related symptoms we're all too familiar with.

For instance, an increase in heart rate and blood pressure can cause discomfort and restlessness. You might also feel a tightening in your muscles and experience headaches which can make those uncomfortable airplane seats feel even worse.

A change in your digestive system is another common stress response. Higher levels of stress hormones slow down digestion as the body prioritizes responding to the perceived threat. This might result in stomach aches, bloating or even changes in bowel habits—in other words, factors that can possibly ruin your adventure.

Speaking of digestion, the relationship between the brain and the gut is important to understand when discussing stress. Called the gut-brain axis, this communication system between your gut and your brain can drastically be affected by stress, potentially leading to bouts of irritable bowel syndrome (IBS) and other gastrointestinal problems.

Ever heard of "stress-eating"? This isn't just a catchy phrase—it's a legitimate response to stress. Under stress, some people find comfort in food, particularly fatty, sugary, or salty foods. As you can imagine, this isn't the best news if you're fighting with weight fluctuation while frequently traveling.

Stress can also affect our sleep patterns. High levels of stress hormones can make it difficult to fall asleep, stay asleep, or even affect the quality of our sleep. And poor sleep can lead to increased levels of cortisol, which can potentially lead to weight gain.

Stress can also weaken the immune system, opening the door to illnesses such as colds, or worse. This is a particular issue while traveling, as you're often exposed to more germs and viruses than you are at home.

Furthermore, stress doesn't just impact us physically—it can also influence our behaviors and emotions. You might feel irritated or overwhelmed, leading to less than positive interactions with others. Not an ideal situation when you're far from home and possibly dealing with language and cultural differences.

So while stress is indeed a natural part of life, it's clear that it can dramatically affect our bodies, particularly in periods of prolonged or frequent travel. By understanding these interactions between your brain and your body, you can better prepare and manage stress reactions, helping to maintain your health while on the road.

In the next section, we'll dive into strategies for remaining calm and aware during stressful travel experiences, mitigating stress's impact on your body. Because knowing how your brain responds to stress is only half of the equation—you've also got to know how to manage it!

Remaining Aware and Calm for the Benefit of Your Body

By this point in our journey, we've delved deep into the science of gut health, the challenges of travel, the significance of circadian rhythms, the role of healthy eating, the importance of exercise, and the impact your brain can have on your body. Now, we're going to focus on an aspect that ties all these factors together—remaining aware and calm for the benefit of your body.

Let's start with the idea of awareness. No, we're not talking about that itch on your nose you just noticed. We mean the deep, intrinsic knowledge of what's going on inside your body. When you're in tune with your body, you can sense when something's off, be it physical discomfort, emotional distress, or irrational cravings. That kind of awareness can alert you to potential problems before they escalate, and help you take proactive steps to maintain optimal health.

Staying calm amidst chaos, on the other hand, asks us to counteract our instinct to panic or stress out. It requires us to avoid getting lost in worries about missed flights, lost luggage, or adjusting to new time zones. Instead, we need to focus on deep breaths and quiet thoughts, serenely dealing with whatever travel throws our way.

Keep in mind that you're not just doing this for mental peace. Awareness and calm can have a direct, positive influence on your physical health, too. When you're aware and calm, your body isn't wasting energy on stress, fear, or anxiety. Instead, it can conserve energy for vital functions, heal faster, and better ward off illnesses.

So, where does one start on the road to becoming more aware and calm? One popular method used by many is meditation. Not just a trendy buzzword, meditation is a time-tested practice that promotes self-awareness and calm. And the best part? It doesn't require any special equipment, and after a little practice, you can do it anywhere, making it a perfect practice for on-the-go travelers.

Another great technique for promoting awareness and calm is mindfulness. This practice encourages being fully present in the moment, concentrating on your breath, the scents surrounding you, the sound of your steps on the ground. By focusing on the present, you become more able to cope with unexpected events, and less vulnerable to reactions fueled by stress or anxiety.

It's also important to take care of your body when attempting to boost your awareness and remain calm. Regular exercise can help with this. Whether it's a brisk walk through the park or a quick yoga session before boarding your flight, exercise can shake off sluggishness, sharpen your mind, and leave you feeling much calmer.

Sleep also plays a crucial role. To achieve a state of calm, you need to make sure you're getting a good night's sleep. That means having a decent bed, a quiet room, and a regular sleep schedule—challenging as that may be when your body's battling jet lag. But by prioritizing sleep, you are ensuring that your body is recuperating, refocusing, and regenerating, allowing you to face each new day with a calm and focused mind.

Another crucial piece of the puzzle is nutrition. What you eat can directly impact your state of mind and calmness. You might have noticed how you feel jittery after too much caffeine or sluggish after eating a heavy meal. The food you choose to consume while traveling can help you maintain mental balance and emotional calm. Try to eat clean, nutrient-dense foods as much as possible. Instead of reaching for that greasy fast-food burger at a layover, munch on some fresh fruits and nuts. You'd be surprised how much this can impact your state of calm.

Staying aware and calm doesn't mean you're immune to travel frustrations—you're simply better equipped to deal with them without spinning into an unhealthy stress-ridden cycle. Think of it like this: when you're aware and calm, the delays and inconveniences of travel are just temporary moments in time, not insurmountable hurdles.

Don't think of it as a chore either. Enhancing your ability to remain aware and calm is a journey—a process of personal growth. Each effort you make, every small victory you achieve, leads you to develop healthier habits while traveling and, quite frankly, while living your life.

Awareness and calm have a holistic impact on your wellbeing. They not only help reduce the physical stress on your body but also promote a positive psychological state. As a result, your body can handle the demands of travel substantially better.

So, after learning about the ways you can stimulate your awareness and encourage calm, are you ready to incorporate them into your traveling lifestyle? Remember, it's not an overnight change. It's a learning curve, and each stride brings you closer to a healthier and happier travel experience. Let's move on next to the practical tips that will help you maintain this balance during travel.

Chapter 7:
Practical Tips:
Maintaining Your Health While Traveling

In the last few chapters, we have peeled back the layers on how traveling impacts various areas of your physical and mental health, from your gut health to the workings of your brain. Now, let's conjure up some practical tips you can build into your travel routine. Let's start with hydration, because simply put, it's a game-changer. Think about it, when you're high in the sky or chugging along on a train, the environment around you isn't exactly replicating earth at ground level. The humidity falls dramatically causing a real threat to your hydration. It's a bit like the desert up there, but without the camels or cacti in sight. Get a good water bottle and keep it refillable. Granules, powders, tabs - whatever it takes to encourage you to drink more, go for it. Speaking of going for it, don't shy away from moving around on those long-haul flights or car rides. Your body's not designed to stay static for extended periods. So, kickstart your circulation with some stretches or aisle walks. Last but not least, managing stress while traveling is as important as packing your passport. It's not a fun fact, but reality is travel can be stressful and that stress has a way of sneakily impacting our physical health. Anything from mindful breathing to light meditation can be a great starting point to deal with this. Now, we got hydration, movement, and stress management. That's check, check, and check. Great practical steps to keep you in check. Don't worry, we won't leave you hanging after take-off, we'll go over more comprehensive plans in the next chapter.

Staying Hydrated

From our last discussion, it's clear that maintaining optimal health while traveling incorporates multiple aspects. One of the most important, yet sometimes overlooked aspects, is staying hydrated. It's easy not to keep track of your water intake when you're on the move, but paying attention to it can make a significant difference in your health and comfort during and after travel.

First things first - why is hydration so crucial, especially while traveling? Your body largely comprises of water, reaching up to 60% in adults! Critical bodily functions, from regulating body temperature to aiding digestion, all depend on us taking in enough water. So whether you're in transit or exploring a new city, staying hydrated should be high on your priority list.

Traveling, particularly flying, leaves you more susceptible to dehydration. The air in the cabin of an airplane is extremely dry, which can lead to dehydration if you don't take in enough fluids. Couple this with the diuretic effects of drinking coffee or alcohol in flight (which, let's face it, many of us do), and you can end up feeling pretty parched.

And no, it's not just about the frequent bathroom trips! Dehydration can take a toll on your body, making you feel tired, impacting your digestion, and making your skin feel dry. If you're traveling to an arid climate, the risk of dehydration gets even higher.

Does water only come from drinking water? Nope! It's not just about guzzling bottles of water. Hydration also comes from the foods you eat. Fresh fruits and vegetables are rich in water content. For example, cucumbers, strawberries, and watermelons are made up nearly of 90% water! Adding these to your travel meals can help up your hydration game and keep bloating in check.

And remember, it's not about drinking a lot of water at once. You should ideally be taking in fluids regularly throughout the day. Frequent sips are better than chugging water all at once. Why? Your body can only absorb a certain amount of water at a time. Consuming large quantities at once will lead to frequent bathroom trips, without necessarily improving your hydration levels.

Water in its pure form is your best friend for hydration. Nutritionists suggest aiming for at least eight 8-ounce glasses of water a day, which is roughly about 2 liters. If you find water too plain, you can spice it up. Infusing water with fresh fruits, herbs or even a dash of lemon can add flavor and make it more appealing to drink, without adding unnecessary calories or sugars.

If you're an avid coffee drinker or can't seem to quit your soda habits, consider swapping out one of your caffeinated or sugary beverages for a glass of water. Not only will this help maintain your hydration levels, but also it could help curb your cravings for unhealthy drinks. It can even help with managing weight fluctuation, which was a concern we addressed in a previous section.

Understanding when your body needs water is also crucial. Thirst isn't always the best indicator of dehydration. Sometimes, our bodies can confuse hunger with thirst. So before you reach out for a snack, have a glass of water. Other signs of dehydration include fatigue, headaches, or a dry mouth or skin. Keeping an eye out for these signs can help you manage your hydration levels better.

Investing in a good water bottle can also be beneficial. Having a bottle handy means you'll likely drink more water. Plus, it's cost-effective and environment-friendly compared to buying disposable plastic water bottles.

If you're traveling to a location where tap water isn't safe to drink, you need to take extra precautions. Always opt for bottled water from reputed brands. Alternatively, carry a portable water purifier or use water purification tablets to ensure that you're drinking clean and safe water.

Lastly, let's debunk a common myth. Drinking alcohol doesn't hydrate your body, it dehydrates it! So if you're enjoying a few drinks on your vacation, make sure you're pairing each drink with a glass of water to balance it out.

Hydration is not rocket science, but it also isn't something you should gloss over, especially while traveling. As we move on, remember our mantra - regular small sips, not big gulps! Drink water throughout your journey, watch your body for signs of dehydration, and enjoy feeling healthier and more energized. Ready to dive deeper into keeping your body moving while traveling? Let's swim right into it!

Regular Movement and Stretching

Traveling often involves lots of sitting, whether it's on a plane, train, or in a car. Transit times can be long and tiring, leaving your body stiff and restless. That's where regular movement and stretching come in. These two factors can make a significant difference to your comfort levels during and after the journey, and also decrease bloating.

Moving regularly and stretching frequently isn't just about feeling more comfortable, though. It's also crucial for maintaining blood circulation in your body. Staying sedentary for prolonged periods can lead to poor circulation which can cause health concerns such as ankle swelling, leg cramps and even blood clots. So keeping your body moving is a matter of health, not just comfort.

When it comes to regular movement while traveling, it's important not to overthink it. Keep it simple. Every hour or so, get up from your seat and walk around for a short while. If you're on a plane or train, this can be as straightforward as walking to the restroom and back. For car journeys, consider making short stops once every couple of hours for a quick walk and stretch.

Don't underestimate the power of doing small exercises in your seat too. Something as simple as rolling your ankles, stretching your neck, or doing a few seat squeezes, where you tighten and release your glutes, can stimulate blood flow and keep your muscles from stiffening up. They're discreet, easy to do, and can provide relief from the discomfort of being stationary for too long.

Stretching your body is another practice to incorporate into your travel routine. Extended periods of sitting can lead to tight and shortened muscles, especially in areas like your hips, back, and neck. Including a few key stretches in your routine can significantly help with this issue.

For your hips and lower back, seated forward bends and knee hugs work wonders. To stretch your neck, gentle neck rolls can be effective. Remember, though, that it's not about pushing your body to the point of pain. Every body is different, so it's essential to listen to yours and do what feels good for it. The goal is to ease discomfort, not cause more of it.

You may be thinking that moving regularly and stretching might draw unwanted attention in public spaces, such as airports or train stations. But the beauty of these activities is that they're subtle and can be done discreetly. Plus, your body's health and well-being should always take priority. Chances are, most people will be too absorbed in their own routines to pay you any mind.

Adding regular movement and stretching into your travel routine also has the benefit of helping you adjust to new time zones. Research has found that light exercise, like walking or stretching, can assist with resetting your circadian rhythm, helping to minimize jet lag.

Regular movement and stretching also indirectly influence your gut health. Physical movement can help regulate your digestion, reduce gas, and decrease constipation and bloating. These are common issues experienced by many travelers and can be alleviated, in part, by staying active and mobile.

Finally, it's worth noting that it's not just those long stretches in transit where regular movement and stretching matter. If you find yourself waiting for hours in airports or train stations, or you're spending a lot of time in meetings or conferences, remember to apply the same principles. Keep your body moving and spend some time stretching. Your body will thank you for it.

In conclusion, incorporating regular movement and stretching into your travel routine can have a multitude of health benefits. Not only can it alleviate physical discomfort and decrease bloating, but it can also improve your circulation, support your gut health, and help adjust your body's internal clock to different time zones. These elements are simple yet potent tools for maintaining your health during travel.

So next time you're on a journey, remember to keep your body moving and take time to stretch. It's all about developing healthy habits that support your body's health and comfort. It might take a bit of intentional effort to get in the habit, but over time, it'll become second nature, and your body will definitely appreciate it.

Stay tuned for more practical tips on maintaining health during travel in the next sections. We'll dive deeper into managing stress during travel, creating pre-travel preparation routines, and more. It's holistic, intentional care for your body that goes far beyond just diet and sleep.

Managing Stress During Travel

Traveling is thrilling. New sights, sounds, exotic foods, and different time zones - it's an ultimate adventure. However, beneath the excitement, there's often stress. Whether it's juggling luggage, rushing to catch flights, or adjusting to different cultures, the stress can be intense. And, remember, your body hears everything your mind says. So, it's essential to curb stress levels to maintain good health and prevent bloating during your travels.

The first tip to successful stress management in transit is all about preparation. Before you start your journey, invest some time in learning about your destination. Understand the culture, know your flight schedules, transit points, and look up essential phrases if they speak a different language. Knowledge, they say, is power, and when you know what to expect, it plays a great role in reducing potential stressors.

Another crucial factor in managing stress is having a detailed yet flexible travel plan. Jot down your daily itinerary, but don't overlook to incorporate some downtime. Remember, a vacation is not supposed to be an endless to-do list, instead, it's an escape from the usual hustle-bustle. Having buffer times and not overscheduling will help you stay flexible when inevitable delays or changes occur.

Next, let's talk about mindfulness. You must have heard about this popular stress-busting technique. Well, it's even more beneficial during travel. Meditation apps can be your best friends when you are on the go. They offer guided mindfulness sessions that can help you stay balanced and calm. It's like having your own tranquil island amid the sea of travel chaos.

Physical activities also play a crucial role in managing stress during your journey. A brisk walk in the morning or a run in the park nearby can stimulate the production of endorphins - the "feel-good" hormones. Not only will this make you feel more relaxed, but it also helps in reducing bloating, a commonly experienced discomfort during traveling.

You might have heard the ancient proverb - laughter is the best medicine. It doesn't only make you feel good, but it also acts as a stress buster. So, ensure that you're making time for fun. Be silly, laugh, meet new people, and create joyful memories.

Another important aspect of managing stress while traveling is to stay connected with your loved ones. Talk to them about your journey, share your experiences, laugh about your blunders. In this digital age, staying connected is easier than ever and works wonders in eliminating travel-induced stress.

While travel offers a delicious spread of luxurious cuisines, it's also crucial to watch what you eat. Consuming healthy, preferably light meals, will not only help you prevent bloating but also boosts your mood. You see, certain foods can increase the brain's serotonin levels, the body's natural feel-good chemical, which then helps reduce stress.

Hydration is another key player in managing travel stress. Remember to keep sipping water during your journey. This simple activity improves digestion, keeps bloating at bay, and also helps you stay alert, thereby reducing the chances of travel-associated stress.

Different time zones can start a daunting fight within your body's internal clock. It's quite important to gradually adjust your body's rhythm before you travel. A gradual shift in sleep routine depending on the time zone of your destination can help minimize the stress associated with jet lag.

Music is a brilliant stress-buster and can be a great travel companion. Carry along your favorite tracks, or try some calming natural music like the sound of rain or waves crashing against the shore. It helps reduce stress by distracting your mind and soothing your senses.

At times, travel can throw the unexpected at you. Luggage can get lost, or a flight might get canceled. It's crucial to remember that such mishaps are part of the journey. Instead of worrying about what's beyond your control, focusing on finding solutions can keep stress at bay.

Aromatherapy is an excellent tool for reducing stress, and it's easy to incorporate into travel. Essential oils like lavender or chamomile can provide calming effects. A drop or two on your pillow can ensure sound sleep.

Finally, take it easy on yourself. Remind yourself that it's okay to make mistakes, it's okay to get lost, it's part of the thrill. You are on a vacation, after all. The goal is to unwind, relax, and enjoy. You deserve it!

In conclusion, travel stress is inevitable, but it's manageable. Employing these simple yet effective techniques during your trips can substantially reduce travel-induced stress and help in maintaining your health. Remember, at the end of the day, traveling is about making fond memories, and stress should never overshadow that beautiful goal.

Chapter 8:
Putting It All Together:
Comprehensive Travel Wellness Plan

On the journey we've been embarking on, we've explored the ins and outs of staying healthy while traveling, from the importance of gut health to the effects of time zones on our internal clock. We've dived into the role brain plays on our body while traveling and the impact of our diet on bloating. Now, let's put these pieces together and create a roadmap. The key is to form a plan that's comprehensive but not overwhelmingly complex. It should begin with diligent pre-travel preparations, including light exercise, hydration, and consuming foods rich in fiber. Once you're on your journey, don't let all your hard work fall by the wayside. Stay mindful of your physical and emotional state, taking time for movement and stress management - whether it's by enjoying local cuisine mindfully or doing a few stretches before bedtime. And finally, give your body the care it needs to recover post-journey. Don't rush back into your routine. Allow your system to adjust and rest up. Remember, maintaining your health is a journey, not a race, especially when traveling.

Pre-Travel Preparations

Before you set foot on a plane, train, or automobile, good preparation is key for a healthy journey. Jumping from one time zone to another, adapting to new foods and cultures, and facing jet lag; all can be stressful. But with the right preparations, you can keep that at bay. Let's take a closer look.

Up there on the priority list should be sorting out your sleep schedule. Try to align your schedule with the destination's time zone a few days prior to leaving. Going to bed one hour earlier each night, for example, can be incredibly beneficial if you're traveling east. Conversely, if you're heading west, it's best to get sleepy a bit later. This trick, in tandem with light exposure adjustment, can prepare your body for the impending shift.

Now onto food. Eating well plays a critical role in maintaining your health during travel. Prior to your departure, consider loading up on high-fiber foods. They help promote a healthier digestive system and can combat bloating. Legumes, berries, avocados, whole grains and broccolis are all great options.

Stay hydrated is another essential factor to keep in mind. Start increasing your water intake a day or two before you leave. Trust me, it's a game changer! But be mindful of your caffeine and alcohol intake. Both can dehydrate your body, which indirectly impacts gut health.

Speaking of gut, maintaining gut health should be in your preparations too. Adding a quality probiotic supplement to your routine could help. It boosts your gut flora, promotes digestion, and helps maintain bowel regularity, making you less susceptible to bloating.

Before you head out, take a closer look at your travel itinerary. Is there ample down-time? Extended periods of movement, while exciting, can be exhausting. Unstructured time helps your brain relax, which in turn reduces your body's stress level.

Next, let's move onto the physical aspect. Aim for regular exercise in the days leading up to your trip. It not only gets you fit but also helps in combating jet lag. It might be helpful to pick out a few simple exercises that you can do during your journey. Walking, stretching, or in-seat exercises are great ways to stay active in transit.

Along with regular exercise, consider doing some relaxation exercises. Moments taken for deep-breathing, meditation, or yoga can significantly reduce stress levels, leading to a healthier body and mind.

Another practical pre-travel tip is to pack wisely. Bring items that bring you comfort or remind you of home. This could be your favorite book, a cozy scarf, or even your favorite snacks. Familiar items can have a grounding effect and play an essential role in self-care.

It's also a good idea to pack a travel wellness kit. Include a water bottle to stay hydrated, healthy snacks to avoid unhealthy airport or gas-station foods, hand sanitizer, sleep mask, earplugs, travel pillow, and natural remedies such as essential oils to combat stress.

Just as important as your physical health is your mental health. Take care of any potential stressors before leaving. This could be anything from wrapping up projects at work to setting up an out-of-office email.

Identify sources of personal stress in your life and try to eliminate or contain them before travel. Managing your stress levels is essential to helping your body maintain its equilibrium during travel.

Last but by no means least, consider getting a health check-up to ensure you're at your peak. It's also the prime time to ask your doctor for any additional health recommendations based on your destination.

By preparing for your journey mindfully, you can create an environment where stress is minimized, sleeping soundly comes more natural, and your gut remains healthily ticking away. These pre-travel preparations ensure you're stepping on your journey with your best foot forward.

Remember, everyone's body reacts differently to travel. Find what works best for you and make any necessary adjustments. Stay open, flexible, and most importantly, enjoy the journey!

Managing Your Health During Your Trip

Here we are, cruising at thirty-thousand feet and you're probably wondering, "So what do I do now?" Let's take a look at how you can actively manage your health while you're on your trip.

Keep Your Hydration Game Strong

The hustle and bustle of travel, especially air travel, can often leave you parched and not even realize it. The dry cab air gets to you and before you know it, you're dehydrated. Always carry a water bottle with you and refill it as needed. Hydrating your body can control bloating and keep your energy levels fueled.

Choose Food Wisely

Remember the food choices we discussed in chapter 4? Stick to those. Avoid gas-producing foods or those with high sodium content. Choose fruits, vegetables and lean proteins. These food choices won't just reduce bloating, they'll also keep you feeling light and energetic.

Keep Moving

Though it may be tempting to sink into that air-plane seat or hotel bed, it's crucial you continue moving. Walk the aisle of the airplane every hour or so, take the stairs instead of the elevator at your hotel or better yet, explore your new surroundings on foot. Movement aids digestion, reducing likelihood of bloating and keeping you fit.

Stay Active, but Don't Overdo It

Nobody wants to spend their whole trip in the gym, but remember the importance of exercise during travel from chapter 5. Try to incorporate some sort of physical activity in your routine. Explore your new location on a bike or go for a swim. But also remember, vacation time is meant for relaxation, don't overexert yourself.

Manage Your Stress Levels

If things don't go exactly as planned, remember it's all part of the adventure. Practice mindfulness and deep breathing to manage stress more effectively. Stress not only makes you feel lousy, it can also upset your gut and lead to bloating.

Listen to Your Body

Your body is pretty good at sending you signals when things go awry. If you're tired, take a break. If you're feeling bloated or uncomfortable, adjust your food choices and water intake. Attuning to these cues can be a big help in keeping you healthy.

Adjust to the Time Zone

As we've discussed in Chapter 3, your body's internal clock can be a tricky thing while traveling. Help yourself adjust by aligning your meal and sleep times with your destination as soon as possible. This synchronization will help reduce bloating, jet lag and general discomfort.

Stay On Top of Your Gut Health

With all the changes in diet, timing, and stressors, your gut may be a little off. Support it with probiotics and make sure you're getting enough fiber, which aids digestion.

Make SMART Goals

It's never too late to plan, even while you're on the trip. Make SMART (Specific, Measurable, Achievable, Relevant and Time-bound) goals for yourself – drink x litres of water, walk y kilometers daily etc. These goals can help keep you focused and in charge of your health.

Moderation is Key

Travel often means trying new cuisines, and that's one of the joys of travel! But try to balance your meals and remember moderation is key. It's fine to indulge a bit though, if only to enjoy local culinary delights!

Don't Forget to Rest

With all this focus on staying active, don't forget to give your body rest. Getting plenty of good quality sleep is essential for recovering from travel fatigue and keeping your digestive system operating optimally.

Protect Your Skin

Don't overlook your skin. Changes in weather and locations can affect your skin. Moisturize regularly and don't forget the sunblock!

By incorporating these ideas and practices, you'll be proactive in managing your health and making the most of your travels. Bon voyage!

Recuperating After Your Journey

Arriving home after a trip, whether it's a quick flight or an extended journey, can often leave you feeling physically drained. Rebound is an essential element of any comprehensive travel wellness plan, and it begins immediately after your expedition ends.

Your body has been through a whirlwind of adaptations, trying to cope with different time zones, diverse cuisines, perhaps unfamiliar physical activity, and other facets of travel. Therefore, it's crucial to give it the time and the gentle treatment it needs to recover fully.

Here, we are going to explore the vital steps to help you recuperate from your journey effectively. Bloating and weight fluctuation are amongst the most common aftereffects of travel, but with the right recovery plan, it's entirely possible to manage these outcomes.

Decompression is the first step in a bounce-back routine. Give your body a day or two to settle down and return to the rhythm of daily routines. Attempting a high-intensity workout or rushing back into a hectic schedule can be counterproductive.

Instead, try engaging in easy exercises, like a brisk walk in your neighborhood or a cooling swim at a local pool to ease your body back into routine movements.

Eating habits play an enormous role in recuperation from travel. Mindful consumption of wholesome foods high in fiber, such as fruits, vegetables, and whole grains, can quickly help reduce bloating.

Moreover, chicken soup is a hydrating and comforting dish to re-energize yourself. The lean proteins it contains can do wonders for your body. Also, try incorporating mushroom broth or seaweed salad, which are known for their detoxifying and anti-inflammatory benefits.

Did you know spicy foods can stimulate your metabolism and assist digestion? Add a bit of ginger or chili pepper to your meals. These ingredients can alleviate symptoms of bloating and stimulate your digestion.

Getting sufficient sleep post-travel is just as crucial for recuperation as exercise and diet. The body repairs and regenerates itself during sleep. Your circadian rhythm could still be adapting to different time zones, so it's crucial to aid it by maintaining a healthy and routine sleep schedule.

Try to get at least eight hours of sleep, and avoid using electronic devices at least an hour before bedtime. Dimming the lights in your room can also help your brain understand it's time to wind down and prepare for sleep.

Remember to hydrate yourself frequently. During travel, we often neglect our fluid intake, leading to dehydration, which can exacerbate fatigue and bloating. Drinking water, herbal teas, or consuming fruits and vegetables with high water content can minimize these effects.

Mental health is equally critical in recuperating post-travel. It's natural to feel a sense of melancholy or stress after returning from a memorable journey. Keep engaging in practices like mindfulness, meditation, or yoga, which can alleviate any post-travel blues.

Lastly, give your body positive reinforcements. Facilitate muscle recovery with a warm bath topped with Epsom salts, schedule a massage, or engage in any relaxing activities you enjoy. Rewards like these motivate your body and aid in quicker recovery.

Remember, the goal isn't just about maintaining health on the move; it's about promoting total wellness throughout your journeys, including the important recovery period once you've returned home. With these tips, you're set to recuperate effectively from your travels and prepare for your next adventure.

Conclusion

Congratulations on making it to the end of your wellness journey in this book. Believe it or not, a passion for traveling does not have to equate to an unwelcome plethora of health-related issues. Making adjustments to our routines, eating habits, exercise routines, and stress management can significantly improve our overall well-being while on the road or in the air.

Remember, your body is a fantastic machine that responds to the way we treat it. If you feed it right, manage stress, keep it hydrated, keep it moving and give it plenty of rest, it'll thank you by keeping up with your wanderlust desires. Your 'gut feeling' about healthy travel is more than just a saying. It's science too, remember everything about gut health and circadian rhythms when planning for your next travel journey.

Ensuring your health and mitigating bloating while traveling are achievable goals. The information provided throughout this guide should empower you to make more informed decisions about your health while traveling. This book doesn't aim to scare you away from your love of travel. Instead, it aims to help you embrace it fully, but in a healthier and more sustainable way. Safe and healthy travels!

Health and Travel Experts to Follow

Being a frequent traveler, especially with concerns over bloating and weight fluctuations, knowledge really is power. And that knowledge doesn't only have to come from books. There's also a wealth of information from experts in the field who've devoted their lives to dissecting the complex interaction between health, travel, and overall well-being. Following these thought leaders can give you valuable tips, new perspectives, and constant reminders to stay on track as you journey across the world.

Firstly, consider **Dr. Michael Breus**, a Clinical Psychologist known as 'The Sleep Doctor'. His in-depth research into the intricacies of sleep greatly aligns with our discussion on circadian rhythms. If you're wondering how to make jet lag less of a monster, he's your guy!

Next on the list is **Luke Jones**, moving us onto the physical fervor of staying fit while traveling. As a movement coach and wellness advocate, he shares accessible exercise tips and techniques, including some that are ideal for travelers confined by limited space or resources.

As for dietary concerns, especially related to bloating, look to **Tamara Duker Freuman**. A registered dietitian specialized in digestive disorders, she's someone whose advice you'd want to gobble down. She often talks about choosing foods for gut health, which can directly impact diet-induced bloating.

When it comes to reducing travel-related stress, there's **Deepak Chopra**. As an advocate of mind-body healing and holistic wellness, his advice can really help your body feel more grounded, mitigating the impacts of constant travel.

And for your overall travel health guide, **Dr. Yael Joffe**, a leading expert in Nutrigenomics, offers fascinating insights into how our bodies react to the challenges raised by frequent traveling. Trust us, her content brings a whole new meaning to 'travel reservations'.

By following these experts, you can blend your love for travel with a drive for healthful living. Their advice can complement the information in this book, giving you a wider spectrum of strategies to personalize your health journey while traveling. Remember, it's not just about avoiding negative health effects, but also maximizing your well-being to fully enjoy every moment of your trip.

Sources With Helpful Travel Tips

Now that we've journeyed through the fundamentals of maintaining your health while traveling, you might hunger for more knowledge and tips to bolster your overall travel experience. Fortunately, there are countless resources that can provide you with more insights, tips, and tricks to enhance your physical health and decrease instances of bloating while you're on the go. To help you further in your journey, we've collected a list of reliable, informative sources.

WebMD's Travel Center: This comprehensive site offers a seemingly never-ending array of articles and advice on every conceivable health concern that can arise during travel. Of particular interest might be their guides dedicated to topics such as "Healthy Travel Foods" and "Staying Healthy On-The-Go".

The Smart Traveler App: Your phone or tablet is presumably almost always with you, and they can be an incredible tool for your health while traveling. The Smart Traveler App can provide easy access to an archive of travel-savvy tips and advice for common health concerns. It also offers insightful videos and articles.

Lonely Planet's Comprehensive Travel Tips: In addition to having a wealth of travel guides, Lonely Planet has resources for healthy travel. They propose advice on eating healthy, how to best recover from long-haul flights, and on battling jet lag effectively.

Nomadic Matt's Healthy Travel Tips:World travel expert, Matt, imparts practical examples and tips from his personal travel experiences. His site includes tips on staying healthy and fit during your travels, maintaining a balanced diet, and reducing stress.

The Healthy Travel Blog: This blog goes deep into the travel experience, exploring many health-related concerns. They tackle topics such as the importance of hydration while traveling, ways to keep your gut healthy, dealing with common travel ailments, managing stress, and more. Their varied range of articles are both specific and practical.

Each of these sources offers a wealth of actionable advice that can help you safeguard your health while you're soaking up new cultures, cuisines, and experiences. Remember, good health is crucial in making the best out of your travels. Now armed with a broader understanding of how your body responds to travel and with these sources in your arsenal, you're even more ready to master your next adventure!

www.ingramcontent.com/pod-product-compliance
Lightning Source LLC
Chambersburg PA
CBHW020358290526
45785CB00005B/2347